YOUR
BEST
DOCTOR
VISIT EVER

12 Proven Strategies
for an Exceptional Visit
with your Doctor

J. Scott Ries, M.D.

Printed in the United States of America
Edited, formatted, and interior design by Kristen Corrects, Inc.
Interior design creation by Bluebird Design Agency, LLC.
Book cover design by D.V. Suresh

First edition published 2017

Ries, J. Scott
Your best doctor visit ever: 12 proven strategies for an exceptional visit with your doctor / J. Scott Ries

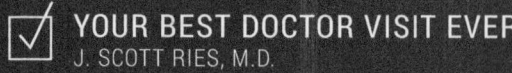

TABLE OF CONTENTS

INTRODUCTION

INTRODUCTION

A friend asked me recently, "Is there anything I can do to have a better visit with my doctor?"

My mind immediately went to Mary.

Just a few days earlier, after giving a talk on health to an engaged audience, I noticed her patiently waiting to speak to me as I greeted a number of attendees.

As she approached, I could tell from Mary's downcast eyes and hesitant stance that something was troubling her.

"I just don't understand it," she confessed. "I really want to discuss these important things with my doctor, but every time I meet with him, I feel so rushed. It's like my mind just goes blank, and I can't remember a thing I wanted to ask!"

Mary and my friend were not the first to ask me for tips on having a better doctor's visit, nor would they be the last. The tandem of increasingly complex health concerns paired with diminishing time with your doctor is a classic setup for frustration.

But there is hope.

With a good plan, a little guidance, and an effective strategy, you can have your best doctor visit ever. You can walk out with your head held high, confident in your understanding and clear on your direction.

I have had the privilege of practicing medicine for over twenty years, including more than 100,000 visits with patients. And I have noted a wide range of how involved people choose to be in their healthcare.

And even as a physician-patient, I've personally experienced many of the same frustrations that you have.

In *Your Best Doctor Visit Ever*, I have distilled the best practices of the most successful patient-doctor encounters into twelve simple strategies.

And with these strategies, you will be equipped to shift from confused to confident as you walk out of your doctor's office with your head held high.

I invite you to dig in, take some notes, and plan your future visit with your doctor. Then let me know how it goes. I'd love to hear your feedback on what you've found most helpful.

Here's to your best doctor visit ever.

CONFIDENT OR CONFUSED?

CONFIDENT OR CONFUSED?

Something has changed.

Gone are the days when putting yourself in the hands of your doctor without a single care, thought, or question is expected simply because of your trust in them. "The era of paternalistic medicine, where the doctor knew best and the patient felt lucky to have him, has ended," wrote Michael Specter in the New Yorker.[1]

And he is correct. Today's vast expanse of healthcare has become too complex, and the demands of exponentially increasing knowledge has healthcare professionals stretched too thin.

Consider the accelerating rate of increase of human knowledge since the time of Christ. Researchers estimate that from year 1 to the year 1500, the sum of human knowledge doubled. Then from 1500 to about 1900, knowledge doubled about once per century. What had previously taken 1500 years, took only 100 years.

Then things really started moving.

Fast forward to the end of World War II, and knowledge doubled at just twenty-five-year intervals. But even that pales to today. With the advent of the Internet, it is estimated that human knowledge now doubles every thirteen months.

But it doesn't end there. IBM estimated that due to the "Internet of things," we will soon experience the doubling of all human knowledge every twelve hours.[2]

So how does this relate to healthcare?

In 1950, the rate of medical knowledge was doubling at a rate of about every fifty years. This was manageable enough for a doctor over the course of a career. What he learned in medical school was generally sufficient, with a few updates here and there.

No longer.

> *From the day a woman conceives her child until the day she delivers, medical knowledge will have doubled…nearly four times!*

By 1990, medical knowledge was doubling at a rate of every seven years. And by 2010, the vast sum of medical knowledge was doubling every 3.5 years.

And it is estimated that by 2020, the total of all of our medical knowledge will be doubling every seventy-three days.[3]

Seventy-three days!

Think of it this way: From the day a woman conceives her child until the day she delivers, medical knowledge will have doubled…nearly four times!

Feel overwhelmed yet? (Hint: So does your doctor.)

But here is where the proverbial rubber meets the road, and where it really matters—knowledge of your health.

So, how did you feel about your knowledge after you walked out of your last doctor's visit? Did you feel confident in your understanding of the precise state of your health? Did you experience great clarity on your pathway forward to a healthier tomorrow?

Or did one of these thoughts creep into your mind?

"What was it she said again about how to take this medicine?"

"Oh no! I forgot to mention the most important part!"

"If only I didn't feel so rushed during our time, I could think more clearly."

"Now I'm totally confused. I don't think I understood a word he said."

If one of these thoughts troubled you, with clouds of doubt and confusion floating through your mind before the hand sanitizer was even dry, don't worry. You are not alone.

There is hope.

Hope for a clear, confident, and rewarding visit with your doctor. One where both you and your doctor leave with a sense of teamwork and alignment. A clear direction in the care of your health.

But it won't happen by chance.

After twenty years of practice, *I've observed twelve strategies that set apart those who are actively engaged in the care of their health* from people who are merely bystanders on the congested highway of medical care.

And what a difference these strategies can make—not only for an office visit, but also for a lifetime of understanding and good health-related decisions.

You are about to discover those twelve strategies, each of which you can employ immediately on your next visit with your doctor.

If you follow these strategies as you prepare for your next appointment, they will guide you into the best mindset possible to take an active role in ensuring your best doctor visit ever.

THE 12 STRATEGIES

STRATEGY

Be an Active Participant in your Healthcare

The person with the most vested interest in your health is…YOU!

Emma Hill, editor of the esteemed medical journal The Lancet, has pinpointed today's reality: "Every patient is an expert in their own chosen field, namely themselves and their own life."[4]

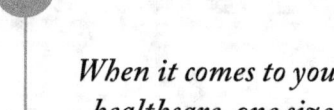

> *When it comes to your healthcare, one size fits none.*

Here is my take. When it comes to your healthcare, one size fits none.

To have the best health possible, you want to make the best health decisions possible. To make the best decisions, you must to have the best understanding possible. To have the best understanding, you must know the facts.

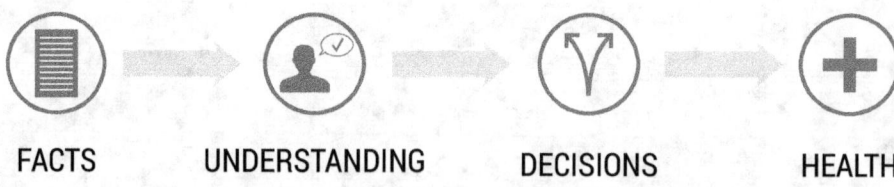

FACTS   UNDERSTANDING   DECISIONS   HEALTH

YOUR BEST DOCTOR VISIT EVER
J. SCOTT RIES, M.D.

Your health is greatly influenced by the decisions you make.

Some of these decisions are momentous:

- *Whether to obtain a colonoscopy to screen for colon cancer*

- *When to seek care for that nagging pain*

- *Whether to fill the prescription given to you*

But most of the daily decisions we make seem much more mundane:

- *Whether to drink water or diet soda with your lunch*

- *Whether to actually do the physical activity you know you need*

- *Whether to schedule screening labs to assess your baseline risk factors*

- *Any many other seemingly small decisions made day after day*

How well informed are you to be able to make the best decisions?

Think of your doctor as your optimal health coach.

I am convinced that people who are the most informed make the best decisions resulting in the best health.

Think of your doctor as your optimal health coach.

Engage with him or her as you make decisions that influence the care of your health. Ask questions. Be honest with your concerns or need to understand your options.

Know your goals. Evaluate your choices. Remain organized in your medical history and medications. These are all important ways to actively participate in your healthcare.

You may have a great healthcare team...*just make sure you are a part of it!*

STRATEGY

#2

Be On Time.

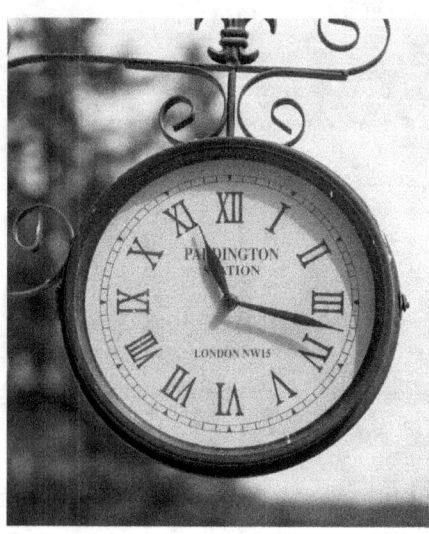

It seems elementary, but timeliness is a necessary courtesy not only for your doctor, but also for other patients with appointments that day.

Arriving just five or ten minutes late can send a ripple effect throughout the day, pushing things further and further behind. Add in the unexpected crises, complicated medical issues, and a barrage of interruptions…and your time in the waiting room can stretch on and on.

Unexpected emergencies can arise for you as well. We know that. No problem, as long as the late arrivals are the exception, not the rule.

Bring a book or a well-charged device to read, and arrive a few minutes early.

Who knows? The person scheduled before you may be late and you might get squeezed in a little early!

YOUR BEST DOCTOR VISIT EVER
J. SCOTT RIES, M.D.

STRATEGY

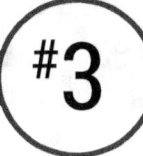

Rank Your Priorities.

It can be challenging to schedule timely visits with your doctor, and you may have several pressing concerns to address while you're there.

However, it's not reasonable to think you can cover all seven items on your list in one visit and still allow your doctor enough time to focus on and evaluate each one thoroughly.

In fact, the quality of your time with your doctor may be inversely proportional to the number of items you want to address. The more issues on your list to discuss, the less the quality (and quantity) of time to devote to them.

To help you stay on track, make a list of your primary concerns and then whittle it down to two or three top issues.

Keep your list of two to three issues in your hand (it's for you, not your doctor), prepare to mention them to your physician, and then move quickly onto Strategy #4!

QUALITY TIME DEVOTED TO ISSUES

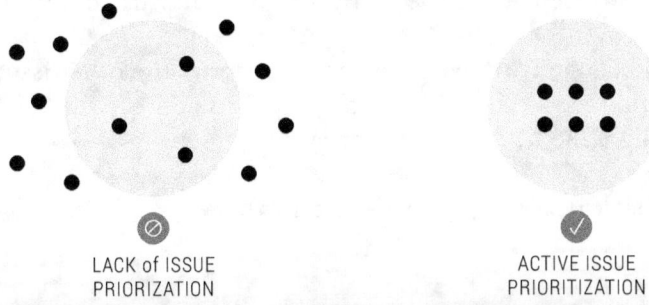

LACK of ISSUE
PRIORIZATION

ACTIVE ISSUE
PRIORITIZATION

STRATEGY

Lead with Your Biggest Concern.

As you present your prioritized concerns, put your biggest concern on the table—first.

I vividly recall one patient who laid out three different concerns at the beginning of our visit, and wanted advice and direction on each.

> *Begin your visit with your primary concern first.*

No problem, it seemed, as I gathered the needed details of each problem, confirmed my suspicion during the examination, and then proceeded to give guidance on each. In fact, I spent a few extra minutes past our allotted time to make sure he was fully informed and on board with the plan to address these relatively minor issues.

And then it happened.

While I was moving toward the door, he energetically offered, "Great! Now that we have those out of the way, the real reason I'm here, Doctor, is because I'm worried about the blood I've been having in my stool."

I wish he had been upfront with his main concern. The other issues were minor and could easily have been postponed to address the potentially life threatening issue he had saved for last.

Begin your visit with your primary concern first.

Leave the less important "Oh, by the way…" concerns for any remaining time at the end, or a future visit if needed. If you're uncertain, it's always appropriate to ask if your doctor is able to address an additional minor concern, or if you will need to schedule a separate visit to do so.

You may be surprised at the answer the gracious question elicits.

STRATEGY

#5

Work Backward—Give the Punch Line First.

When you relate your issue to the staff and your doctor, *start with the punch line.*

What is troubling you the most about your main concern?

Doctors are trained to focus on the chief complaint, so to make the most of your time, let the cat out of the bag at the beginning. Share your biggest concern, and then tell a brief story of the details. It may help to tell the story in terms of these questions:

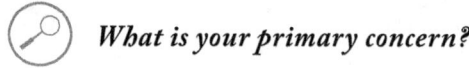 *What is your primary concern?*

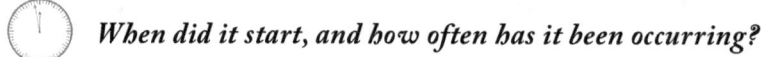 *When did it start, and how often has it been occurring?*

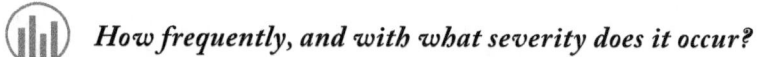 *How frequently, and with what severity does it occur?*

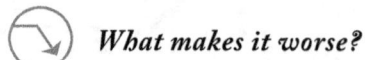 *What makes it worse?*

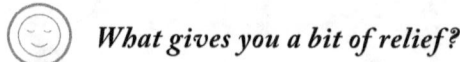 *What gives you a bit of relief?*

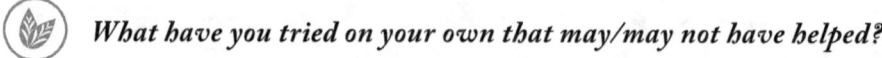 *What have you tried on your own that may/may not have helped?*

☑ **YOUR BEST DOCTOR VISIT EVER**
J. SCOTT RIES, M.D.

Though the details may seem important, resist the temptation to include every chronological nuance of your story.

Work backward.

Pinpoint your concern first, and then relate on your focused story to give the details.

STRATEGY

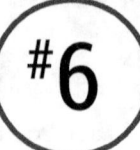

Be Honest.

You cannot embarrass us. Really. We've heard it all. Just be honest.

If you think your embarrassment may be related to your concern and situation, toss it out there. We'll let you know if we think you can overlook it. In similar fashion, if you are not doing something that has been prescribed or recommended, we need to know that as well.

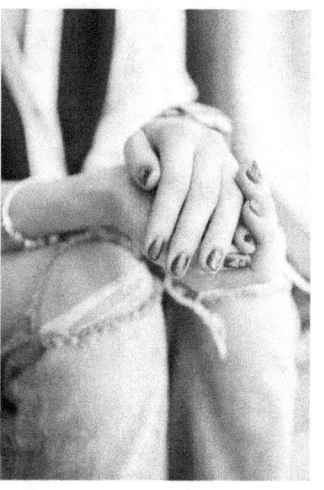

Don't worry, you won't hurt our feelings. Your doctor needs to accurately know the situation in order to best advise you.

If you find you are routinely choosing not to follow your doctor's recommendation, pause and ask yourself why.

- *Could you be taking too much control?*

- *Do you feel like you have a grasp on why your doctor made his or her recommendation?*

- *Is it time to find a different doctor with whom you are more engaged?*

When it comes to your health, honesty is always the best policy.

STRATEGY

#7

Renew Your Medications During the Visit.

If you take prescription medication regularly, take a minute and check your refill status before your office visit. Ideally, you will renew your prescriptions during your visit to the office.

Renewing your prescriptions while still at the office will not only prevent confusion due to medication or dose changes, but will be a win-win situation for:

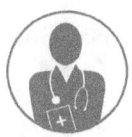

Your doctor and their staff – who will be pleased to meet your needs, and to avoid taking time from someone else's visit to process your refills at a later date.

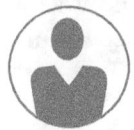

You – who will appreciate the efficiency, and not have to worry about taking your last pill over the weekend, only to discover that you are out of refills.

This simple and often overlooked step can save you hours after your visit, trying to arrange refills between your doctor's office and your pharmacy.

STRATEGY

#8

> ## Document Your Medication and Medical History.

Being organized about the care of your health can be lifesaving. Literally.

Things were moving frantically as soon as the ambulance delivered Robert to the Emergency Room. Though plenty of questions surrounded the situation, one thing was clear: Robert was in trouble. His rapid breathing, altered mental state, high fever, and low blood pressure suggested that he not only had a severe infection, but also had life-threatening sepsis.

Robert needed fast treatment to save his life, including receiving antibiotics immediately. But his family members were not present yet, and we didn't have his prior medical records to assess his allergies.

Thankfully, the paramedic discovered that Robert had a list of his medications and allergies easily accessible in his wallet. Thanks to his list, we learned of his important antibiotic allergies, and avoided giving medication that would make him go from bad to worse.

If you take medications or supplements regularly, make a written list of your medications and carry it with you.

If you are tech savvy, there are also several great apps for your smarthphone that can help you accurately track your medications. A couple of great options include *CareZone (CareZone.com)* and *MyMedications (itunes. apple.com/us/app/my-medications/id478343764?mt=8)* by the American Medical Association.

Make the effort to keep it up-to-date with any changes in dosage or medications, and present it each time you are at the office or hospital.

Feel free to ask your doctor for a printed list of your current medications to compare to your own records. This can be especially helpful if a new medication is prescribed.

The same goes for significant medical problems or surgeries. No need to record each upper respiratory or bladder infection, but we really want to know if you've had your mitral valve replaced and are now on anticoagulants.

Not only will this save precious time, it can avoid confusion or mistakes in keeping up to date on what you are taking, or on what you shouldn't be taking.

STRATEGY

#9

Do Your Homework.

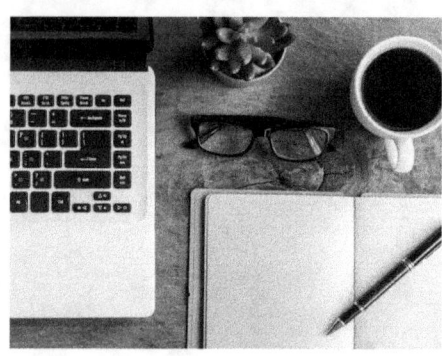

Yes, we know you've already consulted Dr. Google. And no, it doesn't bother us.

But please—*leave the 200 pages of printed articles at home.* We may smile when you hand them to us, but honestly...we won't read them.

Really, we're glad that you are taking the effort to research your concerns. And with information readily accessible online, it makes sense to dig into details. It may help you recognize other symptoms or tidbits of history you had not previously considered.

And if Dr. Eric Topol, cardiologist and one of the most respected researches in medicine, is correct—even bigger changes in store.

In his book *The Patient Will See You Now*, Dr. Topol relates that smartphone-based sensors can now measure just about any physiologic metric previously only measureable by your doctor.

It won't stop there. Soon, many basic labs will be able to be obtained with a simple finger prick, and evaluated through an app on your smartphone.[5]

Until those mobile digital technologies are widely available, there are some websites that are better than others through which you can stay up

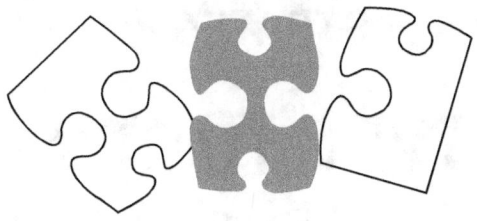

to date on important health topics and to do your research. In addition to health updates at my own www.DrRies.com, here are some reliable sites that I recommend:

- *WebMD.com*

- *MayoClinic.org/diseases-conditions*

- *FamilyDoctor.org*

Once you've done your research, summarize it for yourself and then let us know what you've learned.

Just remember that no matter how much time you spend digging, there will always be one piece of the puzzle you will need to get from us: Context.

There will always be one piece of the puzzle you will need to get from us: Context.

While it is true that your fatigue and headache can be early symptoms of Crimean-Congo hemorrhagic fever, they are much more likely to be caused by the three cups of coffee and two glasses of iced tea washed down by the three diet Cokes you consume daily.

We are here to help you sort through the symptoms and provide the context you need for a correct diagnosis.

So dig in. Study up. Share your findings, concerns, and questions. We will be delighted that you are taking an active role in your health.

STRATEGY

#10

Get Your Labs Before Your Visit.

Activating this strategy can be a game changer.

It can literally transform your visit and the understanding of your state of health from confusion to *confidence and clarity*.

After decades of helping people interpret their lab results, I'm convinced that having your labs drawn and results available before your scheduled office visit is the way to go.

I've observed that patients who obtain their routine lab work prior to their routinely scheduled visit experience the greatest satisfaction and understanding of their progress and state of health.

This may mean an additional trip to the office or the lab a few days before your doctor appointment, but the payoff is worth the additional investment in time.

Having your results in hand during your discussion with your doctor makes tremendous sense. It allows for clarification of the significance of any abnormalities and provides an opportunity for discussion of future goals.

It might take a bit of extra effort, but ask your doctor to order your lab work before your next appointment.

Whether you are planning your next health maintenance physical, or even if you have a visit in a few weeks—leave a message with your doctor requesting to obtain your labs in advance. You'll be glad you did.

"

The payoff is worth the additional investment in time.

STRATEGY

Know Your Numbers.

Nothing says that you are highly engaged in the care of your health more than knowing your numbers.

Regardless of whether you are monitoring metrics for reducing your risk of disease, or are following key indicators of established medical problems, knowing your numbers will empower you for your journey.

In addition to specific monitoring of any medical problems, some important metrics to know and monitor may include your:

- *Weight*

- *Blood pressure*

- *Fasting blood sugar*

- *LDL (bad cholesterol)*

- *HDL ("healthy" cholesterol)*

- *Triglycerides*

- *A1c*

> *Knowing your numbers will empower you for your journey.*

Talk with your doctor about what he or she feels is most important to monitor, and then make sure you track it as well.

Ask for a copy of the results, and *maybe even create your own graph to track your results over time.* The visual will be helpful to highlight your progress at a glance.

STRATEGY

#12

Review Your Visit.

Things can move quickly during an office visit, so it's not unusual to wonder about the specific content or to question the clarity of your understanding later on.

To ensure that you not only receive the guidance you need, but can recall it later, a few simple strategies may help:

- *Bring a trusted friend or loved one to listen in and confirm your understanding*
- *Take brief notes to review later*
- *Discuss your visit with your spouse or close friend*

Finally, summarize the following in writing:

- *Main message and takeaway from your visit*
- *Next action steps you need to take*
- *Additional help you will need (prescriptions, consultations, therapy, etc.)*
- *Follow-up and next appointments needed, and put them on your calendar right away*

Taking the time to read your notes, to discuss your results (to the extent you are comfortable doing so), and to plan your next steps will reinforce what you've learned and experienced during your visit.

Once you've scheduled your next visit, make certain you have the doctor's order for any needed lab tests ahead of time.

To help you plan, track, and record your notes I've created the *Your Best Doctor Visit Checklist.* It is available for you to download—absolutely free. You can find it at www.BestDoctorVisit.com.

BONUS
STRATEGY

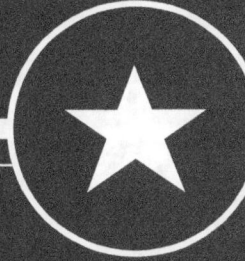

BONUS STRATEGY

Never accept "No news is good news."

Growing up around farms in Indiana, one of my favorite food times of the year was the summer corn season. My mouth still waters when I recall biting into the juicy, sweet, succulent corn on the cob from the farmer down the road.

I remember being a young boy and accompanying my mother to pick up some corn from Farmer John. After exchanging the usual pleasantries, Mom assured Farmer John that a dozen ears of corn would be plenty for today.

As soon as we got home, my job was to shuck the corn as Mom got things ready for dinner. As I dutifully laid out those husked golden treasures, I counted not twelve but thirteen in our dozen.

"Mom!" I exclaimed. "Farmer John gave us too many ears of corn. We told him just a dozen but he gave us thirteen!"

Mom reassured me that all was well in Cornville and that it was Farmer John's habit to give an extra ear of corn, making it a "baker's dozen," as a way of saying thanks to his loyal customers.

So in honor of Farmer John and sweet corn from the heartland, I offer you a bonus "baker's dozen" strategy:

Bonus Strategy: Never accept "No news is good news."

Have you ever walked away from a doctor's office visit, lab visit, x-ray, or some diagnostic test just to be told, "We will call you if anything is abnormal. Otherwise 'no news is good news'"?

> *You are your best health advocate. You are where the buck stops. You are your double-check and your failsafe.*

Just writing those words makes me cringe.

Never, *I mean never*, place your healthcare in the Russian roulette game of "no news is good news."

You are your best health advocate. You are where the buck stops. You are your double-check and your failsafe.

Any time you have a test performed, not only is it *good* for you to know the results, it is mandatory for you to know the results.
Your doctor, lab, specialist, nurse, all mean well. *But they are human.* And humans sometimes let things slip.

I understand that it happens. Just don't let it happen to you.

So the next time you have a lab/study performed, ask this question:

"When will I receive my results?"

It is a very fair and reasonable question, and will elicit one of two responses:

Response #1: "Usually we have the results in three to four days. But if you haven't heard by next Monday, give us a call."

This is an ideal response and one from an office well equipped to keep their patients informed.

Response #2: "Oh, don't worry, we will let you know if there is a problem with your results. If you don't hear from us, everything is fine."

Lights, sirens, and red flags should pop up all over your mind.

But no worries, you are well equipped to respond.

As you warmly smile, graciously but firmly reply:

"Thank you so much, but I always like to follow up on my results regardless of whether or not they are normal. When do you anticipate them back?"

This time you will most certainly get a date. Mark that date down on the *Your Best Doctor Visit Checklist* available as a free download at BestDoctorVisit.com.

If you haven't received the results by that date, phone your doctor's office or send a message through your doctor's online patient portal.

As we discussed in Strategy #11, *Know Your Numbers*, consider keeping a paper or digital copy of the results for personal monitoring and future review.

THE BOTTOM LINE

THE BOTTOM LINE

I have no doubt that your doctor has your best interest in mind.

But there is someone else with even greater interest in the state of your health and your long-term outcomes: *you.*

You are your own best health advocate.

If you don't take an active role as your healthcare advocate and as an investor in your own health, who will?

Within the twelve strategies lies the bottom line:

The more time and effort you invest in the care of your health, the better the health reward you will reap.

The 12 Proven Strategies for an Exceptional Visit with Your Doctor:

#1   *Be an Active Participant in Your Healthcare*

#2   *Be On Time.*

#3   *Rank Your Priorities.*

#4   *Lead With Your Biggest Concern.*

#5   *Work Backward—Give the Punchline First.*

#6   *Be Honest.*

#7   *Renew Your Medications During the Visit.*

#8   *Document Your Medication and Your Medical History.*

#9   *Do Your Homework.*

#10   *Get Your Labs Before Your Visit.*

#11   *Know Your Numbers.*

#12   *Review Your Visit.*

★   *Never Accept "No News is Good News."*

You may find that there are three or four strategies that you want to really focus on immediately. Or, perhaps you are rethinking the entire way you do doctor visits, and you feel a need to incorporate all twelve strategies right away.

Whatever the case may be, these strategies have helped countless patients navigate the turbulent waters of healthcare while bringing clarity to the critical experience of the doctor visit.

Download the *Your Best Doctor Visit Checklist* at www.BestDoctorVisit. com and have hope! A rewarding, satisfying, and exceptional visit with your doctor is not a delirious wish. It is possible. And it is within your reach.

As you follow these twelve strategies, I wish for you your best doctor visit ever!

LEARN MORE

ACKNOWLEDGEMENTS

When I was in medical school, a wise and learned physician once advised me that of all the instructors I would have in my lifetime, my greatest teachers *would be my patients.*

And he was correct.

I am ever grateful for the lessons, perspectives, insights, and encouragement I've received from my patients over the years. You have taught me well, and helped me to remember the reason why I do what I do.

Before publishing this book, I had great feedback and input on the "beta version" from supportive friends and colleagues who have taken their own transforming steps to better health through the iFactor Course.

My thanks go out to:

Judy Bowen	*Bob Ries*	*Donna Parrott*
Terrie Jones	*Chad Frye*	*Sandy Smith*
Lainey Pfister	*Michael McLaughlin*	*Chad Griffin*
Jill Burke	*Melanie Rolley*	*Celeste Pechette*
Jim Lin	*Rosie Francis*	*Sharon Wilson*
Valarae Pfister	*Kevin Miles*	*Ken Jones*
Jeannette Dessaigne	*Scott Santee*	*Connie Phillips*
Gina Lawrence	*David Ginsburg*	*Barb Zazas*

Without the superb editing skills of Kristen Hamilton, Kelli Williams, and Randy Gilmore, this book would have looked much different (and not in a good way!). Wonderful work, friends. You are each a blessing!

What joy to have the love of a supportive family. I could not imagine life without my wonderful wife, Jodi, and our three great kids, Grace, Lauren, and Jason. I love you dearly!

And last and most, the person to whom I am forever grateful is the Great Physician himself. As one sign famously heralds at the entrance of a mission hospital in Kenya, we physicians treat...but it is Jesus who heals.

SOURCES & REFERENCES

[1] Specter, Michael. "The Operator." The New Yorker, February 4, 2013. http://www.newyorker.com/magazine/2013/02/04/the-operator

[2] "The Toxic Terabyte," IBM Global Technology Services, July 2006. http://www.935.ibm.com/services/no/cio/leverage/levinfo_wp_gts_thetoxic.pdf

[3] Jensen, Peter. "Challenges and Opportunities Facing Medical Education." Transactions of the American Clinical and Climatological Association 122 (2011): 48-58.

[4] Hill, Emma. "Smart Patients." The Lancet Oncology 15, no. 2, 140-41.

[5] Topol, Eric J. The Patient Will See You Now: The Future of Medicine Is in Your Hands. New York: Basic Books, 2015. Print.

YOUR BEST DOCTOR VISIT EVER
J. SCOTT RIES, M.D.

iFACTOR HEALTH

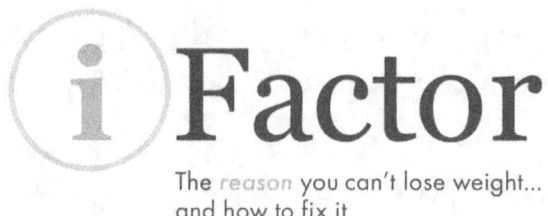

The *reason* you can't lose weight...
and how to fix it.

Do struggle with any of these common problems?

- *Frustrated with your weight?*
- *Can shed a few pounds, but then always regain them?*
- *Run out of energy too early during the day?*
- *Sleep poorly?*
- *Difficulty concentrating at work or at home?*

If you can say yes to any of these symptoms, it is likely you have a problem with your iFactor.

Learn how you can join the community of hundreds of others who have fixed their iFactor and transformed their life.

There is hope to not only lose weight, but *to keep it off* for the long term—and feel better than ever!

Learn more at *iFactorHealth.com*

BEST DOCTOR VISIT WORKSHEET

Get your free *Best Doctor Visit Worksheet* to help you organize yourself for your best doctor visit ever.

This helpful worksheet helps you to prepare for your visit, stay on track during your visit, and prompt you to action afterward.

Download your free Best Doctor Visit worksheet at *BestDoctorVisit.com* today!

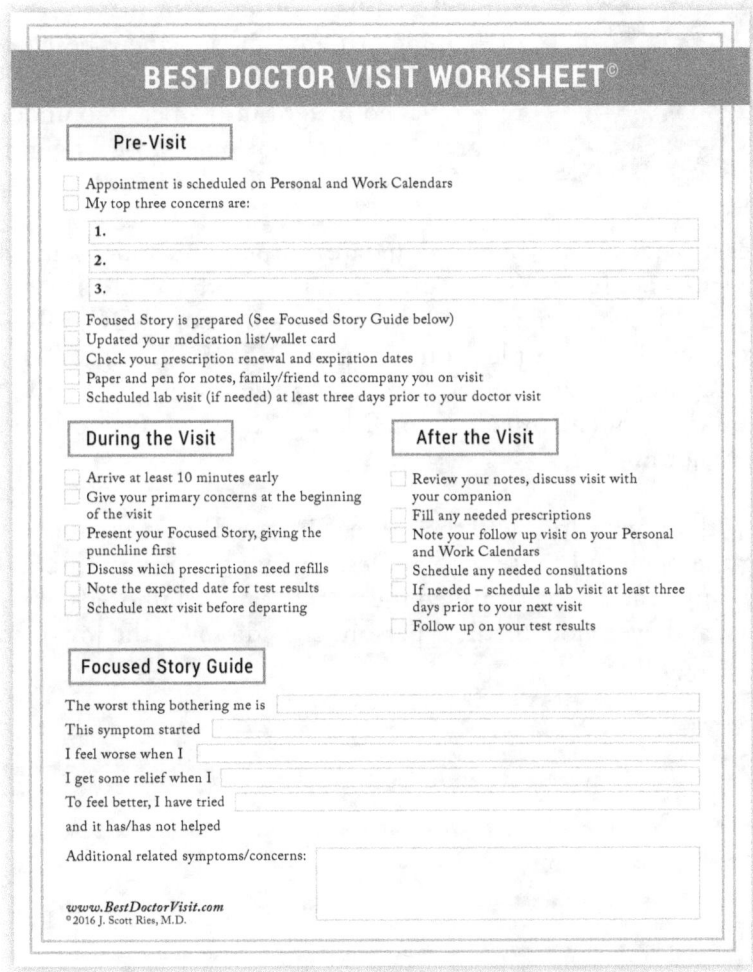

YOUR BEST DOCTOR VISIT EVER
J. SCOTT RIES, M.D.

ABOUT THE AUTHOR

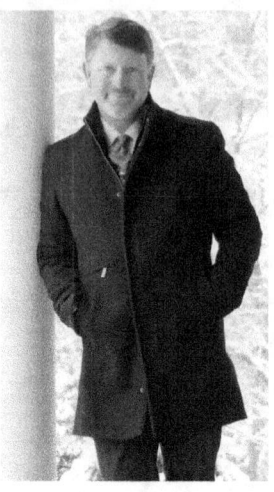

Dr. J. Scott Ries is a board certified Family Medicine and Emergency Medicine physician, and founder of *iFactor* Health. A gifted communicator, Scott specializes in helping people make sense of today's complex medical issues in a way that is clear and understandable.

His career has spanned academic, research, and clinical responsibilities over his twenty years of helping patients pursue their best possible health. He has compiled decades of experience, research, and insight into an easy to understand program to help people lose weight and transform their health—the *iFactor Course*.

Dr. Ries provides timely medical updates through his blogs and podcast at *DrRies.com*. He is also heard on major media outlets across the country, and has been featured in interviews for Fox, NBC, CBS News affiliates, as well as multiple print sources such as *The Lancet, AMA News, Today's Christian Doctor,* and others. He is the host of a weekly health commentary segment broadcast on Moody Radio Network stations in several major markets.

Along with his wife, Jodi, and their three kids, Dr. Ries is passionate about serving the poor and those who are less fortunate through international medical missions. He has traveled the world, leading hundreds of doctors, students, and even non-medical personnel to discover the joy of serving and blessing others.